From Boomers to Zoomers:

Vintage Wisdom Meets Beta Energy

The Timeless Journey:

Redesigning Age in a World Obsessed

with Youth, Filters and Avocado Toast

Ingrid-Astrid von Anhalt

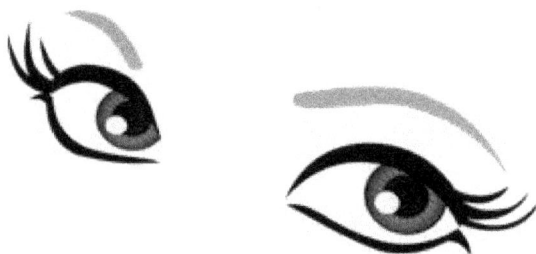

Disclaimer

This book is a work of advice, guidance, information and opinion.

Table of Contents

Dedication

To everyone who has ever been told they are "too old" and responded with a laugh or a perfectly timed emoji.

To the brave souls who age out loud, wrinkles, wisdom and Wi-Fi passwords intact.

To those redefining what it means to grow older in a world that still thinks youth comes with a ring light and a side of smashed avocado.

. . . . This one is for you.

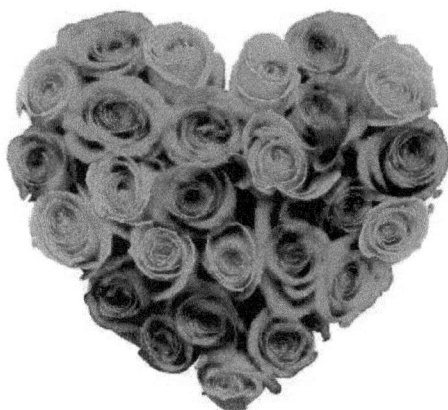

Acknowledgement

I would like to express my sincere gratitude to everyone who has supported me on this journey. To my friends who shared their thoughts about aging with me openly and honestly and for their unwavering encouragement, I am deeply thankful.

I also want to thank the age discriminators. Without having witnessed your doubts and prejudices, I might never have embarked on this journey of writing. In many ways, you gave me the push I needed and, at times, even the comic relief to see the lighter side of it all.

About The Author

Ingrid Astrid is an Australian author whose work delves into various layers of culture and the ever-evolving landscape of relationships. With a passion for writing, she creates uplifting and often provocative content that challenges social norms and invites readers to think differently about love, identity, age, power and belonging.

She is particularly interested in disrupting conventional thinking and inspiring meaningful reflection, encouraging her readers to question the status quo and embrace a different perspective on life. After a successful career in the commercial sector, she has exchanged the boardroom for a more expressive life, where her commitment to new approaches continues to thrive.

Introduction

Why is so much of life dictated by age, as if the moment you hit a certain number, an invisible gong sounds and you are expected to trade in your dreams for knitting needles, or worse, start getting excited about cruise brochures and vitamin organizers? Who came up with this bizarre timeline, anyway?

By 30, you are supposed to have life all figured out. By 50, you are meant to calm down: no more skinny jeans, no loud opinions, and definitely no new tattoos. And by 70? Apparently, you are expected to quietly disappear into a beige cardigan, take up birdwatching, and slowly lose your cognitive sparkle until your brain resembles a ripe banana.

But here is the plot twist: age is not a script. It is not a forecast or a finish line. It is just a number, not some dusty instruction manual marked "appropriate behavior by decade." Should not life be based on who we are, how we feel and not on what year we were born?

Too often, age is used as a lazy shortcut for judging someone's relevance, value or ability to operate a smartphone without panicking. Sure, there are a few exceptions. Age still matters when applying for things like pensions, tax breaks or senior discounts (because who does not love a good discount?). And also, there is a valid reason to state age when it is relevant for legal matters, passports, last wills, licenses, and yes, doctors need to know your age unless you want your symptoms diagnosed via clairvoyance. For minors, proof of age for permissions is essential. But outside of those necessary bits, can we please stop treating age like a universal life instruction manual?

You are not expired; you are just experienced. And that is worth a lot more than a number on a form.

However, frivolous and unessential age requests need to be ignored, as they are more about social norms than necessity. You do not need to share your age at job interviews unless directly relevant (for example, a child actor in an age-based role). In social settings your worth does not come with a number tag. Age is unessential when it comes to online interactions, gym memberships, dating profiles and even shopping. We should challenge those defaults.

Why are people who are no longer "younger" spoken to as if they have just wandered off from the bingo hall and forgotten their own name? Given the way society talks to more mature individuals, one would think they are moments away from confusing the TV remote for a cell phone. It is both insulting and unintentionally hilarious. Mature people did not survive dial-up internet, questionable fashion trends and actual growing up just to be treated like they cannot grasp basic notions and principles.

Suddenly, the same people who once juggled mortgages, investments, and launched three kids through university like fiscal trapeze artists are now treated as if they need a financial babysitter. One minute you are trusted with a six-figure portfolio and the next, a bank teller is squinting at you like you just asked to withdraw your life savings to invest in pirate gold.

Want to access your own money? Be prepared for a pop quiz. "Why do you need it?" they ask, as if you are planning to blow it all on magic beans and a one-way cruise to the moon. Heaven forbid you show interest in cryptocurrency. Mention Bitcoin and suddenly the fraud department materializes like the financial version of the Avengers, threatening to freeze your account before you can say "blockchain." It is like you have gone from respected financial wizard to time-traveled relic who wandered out of a Victorian time capsule marked fragile: keep away from banking.

Apparently, age brings wisdom unless you are at the bank. Then it just brings suspicion, paperwork and a polite suggestion that you stick to crossword puzzles and government bonds.

And then there is the government, quietly peeking over your shoulder. Especially when it comes to driving. Depending on which state or territory you live in, once you reach a "mature" age, your ability to drive is suddenly under the spotlight as if you have woken up one morning and forgotten how to steer without mowing down a letterbox or parking diagonally across four bays.

Never mind the decades you have spent behind the wheel, expertly navigating traffic, dodging potholes and surviving family road trips with nothing but a thermos and a prayer. Now you must prove you can still handle a vehicle without transforming into a hazard on wheels. Apparently, experience counts for less than your ability to read a number plate at twenty paces and not mistake the accelerator for the radio.

Maybe, just maybe, we could stop assuming that turning a certain age means your brain has gone into sleep mode. Not everyone over 70 is a menace in motion; some individuals are still better drivers than half the P-platers out there texting while merging. How about we ditch stereotypes and give people a little credit before we take away their keys and hand them a bus timetable?

So, buckle up. Age discrimination is alive and well. Society's attitude leaves much to be desired while continuing to pretend that youth comes with irresponsibility and mature-aged wisdom comes with an expiry date.

In a world where anti-wrinkle creams sell faster than lottery tickets, turning 50 is treated like a moral failing. But guess what? People in their 60s, 70s, and beyond are out here running marathons, launching apps and falling in love again (and again, sometimes on purpose). Maybe the secret is not in chasing youth, but in mastering the fine art of not giving a damn. Collect memories, not candles. Want to start a podcast at 65 ranting about how children do not know what a fax machine is? Go ahead, that is content gold. Want to take up salsa dancing at 80 or cha-cha really slow? Do it. Once you stop fearing birthdays and start celebrating survival, life gets tastier. Age is not a deadline; it is a privilege.

Depending on where you live, aging is either a badge of honor or a sign that your software is due for an update. In many Western countries, getting older is seen as a slow fade into irrelevance. Knees creak, the fashion world forgets your existence, and society pretends you have vanished unless there is a stairlift commercial to film. This has birthed the bizarre assumption that if you have a pension card, you must also be confused by Instagram, allergic to emojis and deeply suspicious of Artificial Intelligence (AI). Ageism spreads faster than gossip at a high school reunion, yet these same "old people" are the ones who built the very technology younger folks now call "vintage."

In many Eastern cultures, aging is like finally being promoted to family CEO. Gray hair is a crown of wisdom, not a reason to panic-buy hair dye. Elders are revered as sacred story-keepers, parenting pros and walking history books, and they probably know where the emergency cash is hidden. In these places, Nana is not shipped off to the retirement village; she is running the house, the kitchen and possibly the black-market spice trade.

Religion, too, treats aging with flair. In Hinduism, old age is sacred, not just an excuse to complain about how loud the music is. Meanwhile, in hyper-youth societies, screen time is reserved for anyone under 30 who can dance without pulling a hamstring.

The media swings wildly. Sometimes we get glorious, silver-haired badasses. Other times, older characters are portrayed as fragile, mumbling and losing arguments to revolving doors. If aliens watched our commercials, they would assume everyone over 65 is terrified of falling over or being unable to locate the toilet. That is not aging, that is bad marketing.

Here is the punchline: aging is not a crisis; it is a character arc. Around the world attitudes toward aging vary wildly, but one truth remains, growing older does not mean fading out. It means turning up the volume on your personality and maybe misplacing your reading glasses in the fridge while doing it.

Let us celebrate the fabulous weirdos who have lived long enough to say "I told you so" and have the receipts to prove it. Let us rewrite the narrative. Age does not mean less sparkle, it means more seasoning. So go ahead, wear leopard print, learn Portuguese, flirt shamelessly, and remember, you are not getting old, you are just getting more you. Because in the end, age is just a number, not a life sentence, and sass, smarts, and a sense of humor are forever.

Chapter 1:

The Concept of Age

Rethinking the Numbers:
With a Wink and a Wobble

In today's number-obsessed world, age has become the most overused shortcut to judge someone, right up there with zodiac signs and the size of your coffee order. You are either too young to know better or too old to be out in public unsupervised. Apparently, if your birth year starts with the wrong digit, society starts whispering behind your back like you just walked into a high school cafeteria wearing Crocs and confidence.

But here is a wild idea: what if age is not a countdown to irrelevance but a delicious cocktail of life experience, accidental wisdom, emotional mileage, and yes, a few tragic haircuts that are now retro anyway?

The obsession with age has produced more stereotypes than reality TV. You are expected to act your age, dress your age and even dream your age. Who came up with that nonsense? Likely someone who thinks 50 is "basically elderly" and that TikTok is a credible news source.

If we tossed out these dusty old rules, we would create a world where a 70-year-old can launch a business empire, and a 50-year-old can learn to skateboard. Pride optional, helmet highly recommended.

And do not get me started on how systems treat age. Workplaces, social clubs, even dating apps act like your birthdate determines your ability. Last time I checked, creativity did not come with an expiry date. Inspiration does not care if you have reading glasses and a loyalty card at the pharmacy. The real magic happens when fresh enthusiasm meets well-aged cunning. Innovation loves a good cross-generational brainstorming session, especially if there is cake.

Getting older is not a tragedy; it is a glow-up with better stories. Every decade is a new chapter, and let's face it, some of us do not get truly interesting until at least chapter five. Whether it is switching careers, writing your memoirs or finally learning to tango without falling into the pot plant, there is no age limit on joy. Aging should come with a permission slip that says: "Live out loud, wrinkles be damned."

So yes, let us rethink the numbers. Rip up the calendar. Your age is just your Earth mileage. It says nothing about how alive you are and that is entirely up to you.

For reasons known only to the mysterious forces of societal nonsense, we still treat age as if it is the cosmic receipt for "years lived," with no mention of the plot twists, scandal or spontaneous dance parties that happened along the way. Judging someone by their age is like judging a book by how many pages it has instead of whether there is a love triangle, a surprise villain or a scene-stealing parrot inside.

Age is not about creaky knees, it is about the stories we carry. It is not just a date on your driver's license; it is a patchwork of "remember when?" and "I still might." Yes, you might still dye your hair pink. You might still run away with a jazz band. You might still figure out how to use Dropbox without crying.

In a world where anti-wrinkle creams sell faster than lottery tickets, turning 50 is treated like a moral failing. But guess what? People in their 60s, 70s, and beyond are out here running marathons, launching apps and falling in love again (and again, sometimes on purpose). Maybe the secret is not in chasing youth but in mastering the fine art of not giving a damn.

Collect memories, not candles. Want to start a podcast at 65 ranting about how children do not know what a fax machine is? Go ahead, that is content gold. Want to take up salsa at 80? Cha-cha really slow, cha-cha, nonetheless. Once you stop fearing birthdays and start celebrating survival, life gets tastier. Age is not a deadline; it is a privilege.

Depending on where you live, aging is either a badge of honor or a sign that your software is due for an update. In many Western countries, getting older is seen as a slow fade into irrelevance. Knees creak, the fashion world forgets your existence, and society pretends you have vanished unless there is a stairlift commercial to film. This has birthed the bizarre assumption that if you have a pension card, you must also be confused by Instagram, allergic to emojis and deeply suspicious of AI.

Ageism spreads faster than gossip at a high school reunion. Yet these same "old people" are the ones who built the very technology younger folks now call "vintage."

In many Eastern cultures, aging is like finally being promoted to family CEO. Gray hair is a crown of wisdom, not a reason to panic-buy hair dye. Elders are revered as sacred story-keepers, parenting pros and walking history books and they probably know where the emergency cash is hidden. In these places, Nana is not shipped off to the retirement village, she is running the house, the kitchen and possibly the black-market spice trade.

Religion, too, treats aging with flair. In Hinduism, old age is sacred, not just an excuse to complain about how loud the music is. Meanwhile, in hyper-youth societies, screen time is reserved for anyone under 30 who can dance on YouTube without pulling a hamstring.

The media swings wildly. Sometimes we get glorious, silver-haired badasses. Other times, older characters are portrayed as fragile, mumbling, and losing arguments to revolving doors. If aliens watched our commercials, they would assume everyone over 65 is terrified of falling over or being unable to locate the toilet. That is not aging; that is bad marketing.

Here is the punchline: aging is not a crisis; it is a character arc. Around the world, attitudes to aging vary wildly, but one truth remains. Growing older does not mean fading out. It means turning up the volume on your personality and maybe misplacing your reading glasses in the fridge while doing it.

Let us celebrate the fabulous weirdos who have lived long enough to say "I told you so" and have the receipts to prove it. Let us rewrite the narrative. Age does not mean less sparkle; it means more seasoning.

So go ahead, wear leopard print, learn Portuguese, flirt shamelessly, and remember, you are not getting old, you are just getting more you. Because in the end, age is just a number, and sass, smarts, and a sense of humor are forever.

Technology is getting in on the act, too. Wearables now track our heart rates, sleep cycles, stress levels, and even our mood swings during back-to-back Zoom meetings. It is like having a personal trainer, wellness coach, and an overly involved aunt all rolled into one, strapped to your wrist. With so much real-time feedback, staying healthy no longer requires guesswork or a crystal ball.

Aging, once seen as a slow shuffle toward slippers and early dinners, is fast becoming a thrilling second act filled with energy, curiosity, and yoga poses that make you question your flexibility and your life choices.

Of course, there is also the classic debate: "nature versus nurture." Did you inherit your grandfather's cholesterol or is that just the six donuts talking? Genetics and environment are the co-authors of your life story. Think of your DNA as the blueprint and your environment as the wildly unpredictable interior designer. Your genes might hand you a head start or a few unfortunate surprises, but how you live in that body, day by day, shapes how you age. A toxic environment can take even great genes on a detour, while a supportive one can rewrite a family history of heart disease with kale smoothies and laughter therapy.

Living in sunshine, eating Mediterranean-style meals, and dancing like no one is judging your moves, these things matter. Genetics may load the gun, but lifestyle pulls the trigger. And while you cannot change your family tree, you can absolutely prune it and decorate it with disco balls. So, if someone credits their youthful glow solely to DNA, feel free to smile and say, "Sure, but my spinach smoothies and 10,000 steps a day are putting those genes to work."

Aging is not about counting the years, it is about making the years count. It is not just in your chromosomes, it is in your kitchen, your playlists, your friendships and your fabulous refusal to act your age. We are all delightful mashups of inherited quirks and lived experiences, strutting through the decades in whatever shoes our feet will tolerate. And that is aging with flair, with science and with a healthy dose of sass.

And let us not forget the power move in all of this: reflection. In a world full of noise and shiny distractions, taking time to pause is practically revolutionary. Whether it is journaling, meditation, or just staring into space while pretending to do yoga, reflection helps connect the dots between where you have been, where you are, and where you might want to go next (even if it is just to the refrigerator). It helps you hear yourself amid all the shouting and maybe figure out that you are not too old for anything, just too wise to waste time on things that do not matter.

Reflection is where the magic happens. It is how we realize we have grown, how we make peace with what did not go to plan, and how we start crafting a story that feels less like a script and more like a wild, glorious improv show. And when we share these insights, whether over wine, coffee or an interpretive dance, we bridge the gaps between generations. We remind each other that aging is not about shrinking into invisibility, it is about standing taller in your truth, even if your knees creak when you do it.

So go ahead, change it up, laugh loudly, reflect deeply, and say yes to the detours. Life is not about staying the same. It is about becoming more YOU with each delightful, unexpected, and slightly nonsensical chapter.

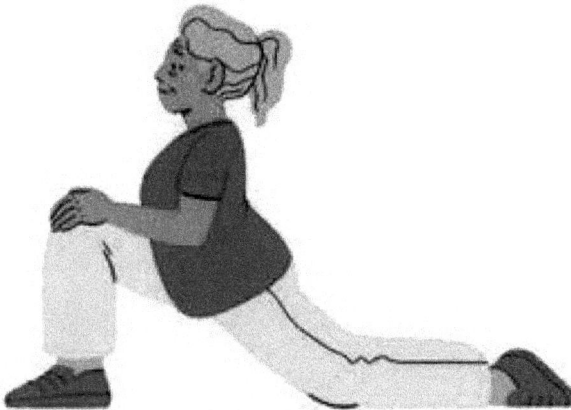

Stay fit so you can
chase your
dreams.......and the ice
cream truck

Chapter 2:
The Science of Aging
Biological vs. Chronological Age

Age is that rickety old tightrope we are all walking, but as it turns out, there is more than one rope. We have chronological age, which is the number of birthdays we have celebrated; the age that decides when we can vote, drive or receive suspiciously cheerful brochures about funeral insurance. It is the number of candles that eventually become so numerous that we either switch to a number candle or risk a small blaze on the cake.

Then there is biological age, the sassier, more temperamental sibling. It does not care how many calendars you have flipped. It is more interested in how you treat your body, how well you sleep, whether you hit the gym or hit the snooze button, and if your dinner choices lean toward salad or deep-fried regret. Biological age is the age your knees whisper to you when they sound like bubble wrap, or when you leap out of bed like a caffeinated gazelle. Two people might be the same age on paper, but one is training for marathons while the other is becoming one with their couch. It is not about the candles; it is about how brightly you are still burning.

Unfortunately, society tends to treat chronological age like an expiration date. Past 50, it seems you are expected to start organizing your will and mastering Sudoku. But when we shift our focus to biological age, aging gets a much-needed makeover. Being 70 with the energy of someone half your age is not magic, it is maintenance (and maybe a splash of green juice). It is about challenging tired stereotypes and making space for a life that is not just longer but richer. Wrinkles become experience badges, not warning signs. The goal is not just to survive longer, it is to thrive louder.

And we are in luck because science is catching up with this new mindset. Longevity research is evolving faster than you can say "anti-aging serum." Scientists are diving deep into our cells, decoding the mysteries of what makes us age and, more importantly, how to do it with style. Words like "cellular senescence" and "telomere shortening" might sound like something out of a sci-fi film, but they are the keys to understanding why some people seem to be surfing into their nineties while others are slumping into their sixties.

It turns out that our DNA holds some promising secrets. Researchers are studying centenarians who still garden and attend dance classes, hoping to bottle their biological magic. But while your genes may set the stage, your lifestyle writes the script. You cannot binge-watch your way to 100. A healthy life still calls for mindful choices: nutritious food, movement, mental calm, and the occasional laugh that shakes your core (and possibly your bladder).

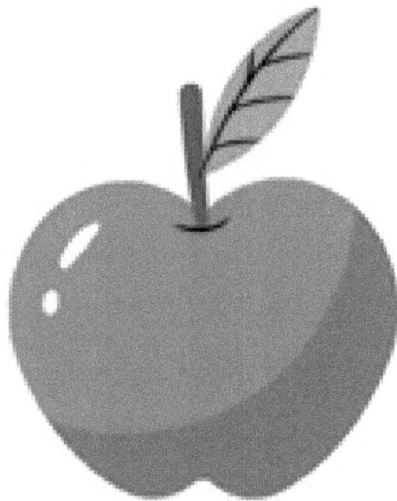

......good things
ahead......

Chapter 3:
The Emotional Landscape of Aging
Embracing Change

"Change" that cheeky little life guest who never RSVPs. One minute you are cruising along with your cappuccino and familiar routine, the next you are being asked to meditate, eat fermented cabbage, and understand cryptocurrency. Still, embracing change is like ordering off the secret menu of life. It is weird at first, possibly spicy, occasionally enlightening, but always memorable.

Society loves to stamp us with a use-by date, as if evolution shuts down after 50. But guess what? You can absolutely dye your hair purple at 65, take up break dancing at 70, or finally admit that your cousin's fruitcake tastes like potting mix.

Life is not a straight, well-lit highway; it is more like a bumpy game of snakes and ladders with occasional glitter cannons and the odd existential pothole. And every plot twist is a chance to reinvent yourself, acquire a fresh look, set new goals, maybe even a surprising new obsession with oat milk. The older we get, the more change feels like being told to swap your coffee for celery juice. But leaning into the unknown? That is where the good stuff lives.

You do not have to start skydiving, unless of course that is your thing but maybe you try paddle boarding, join a pottery class, or (gasp) finally delete your ex's cellophane number. These small rebellions whisper to the universe, "I am still evolving, thank you very much."

Adaptability has become a superpower in a world where apps update more often than the weather. It is not just about keeping up with Instagram reels, but about staying curious, staying open, and possibly being a little cooler than our children are willing to admit. The more we step out of our comfort zones, the juicier life gets. You meet unlikely friends, try foods you cannot pronounce, and start having oddly passionate debates about which brand of oat milk truly froths best.

Of course, all this flexibility does not just happen by accident. It is backed by something solid: wisdom and resilience. Think of them as the deluxe internal suspension system that helps us navigate life's potholes. Wisdom is not just about knowing stuff, it is about knowing what really matters (spoiler alert: it is rarely what is trending). And resilience is that bounce-back juice, the invisible trampoline beneath all those "What now?" moments.

You do not earn these qualities by staying safe in your bubble. They are built through trying, failing, getting up, dusting yourself off, and maybe laughing while you do it. It is falling flat on your face with grace and turning it into a story that makes people snort-laugh at dinner parties. Together, wisdom and resilience become your secret sauce, a blend that helps you sidestep society's limited view of aging and say, "Actually, I am just getting started.."

Chapter 4:

Social Constructs of Age

Ageism: A Wrinkle in Society's Logic

Age is a funny thing. One minute you are the youngest in the room, the next you are being offered a senior discount you did not ask for, and you are not sure whether to be offended or thrilled. Society, bless its confused little heart, has turned age into a bizarre game of bingo where nobody wins and everyone is either "too young to know anything" or "too old to still be trying."

Apparently, once you are no longer wearing glitter eyeshadow or doing keg stands, you are expected to fade quietly into a recliner and start shouting at the TV. But ageism is not just a playground for rude relatives and bad sitcoms. It is baked into the very walls of our workplaces and served daily by the media with a side of condescension.

You have seasoned professionals being nudged toward the exit like expired yogurt, while younger folks are patronized as if they were born yesterday (which, to be fair, they kind of were, but still). Heaven forbid, a 25-year-old have a good idea or a 65-year-old learn how to use Discord. Somehow, we have collectively decided that innovation and experience cannot sit at the same table, probably because we are too busy arguing over who gets the auxiliary cord.

If the media, especially TV, were our only guide, people over 50 would be either confused, cranky, or quietly crocheting in the background. Meanwhile, the under-30s are portrayed as either genius disruptors or exhausted zombies who cannot put their cellphones down long enough to form a thought. Reality check: the world is full of 70-year-olds discovering digital art, launching businesses, and generally putting their younger counterparts to shame. And yes, there are some twenty-somethings who do read books made of paper and can change a flat tire without asking Google.

We need better stories. We need the ones that feature the 80-year-old learning to DJ, the teenager starting a nonprofit, the 60-year-old discovering pole dancing, and the Gen Zs teaching Grandma how to code. Imagine the possibilities when you put vinyl collectors and TikTokers in the same room. Sure, there may be a mild debate over whether "LOL" means "lots of love" or "laugh out loud," but that is half the fun. Eventually, someone is doing the worm, someone is sharing wartime recipes, and everyone is realizing that "generation gaps" are mostly made up by people who sell anti-aging cream.

When did we start treating age like a use-by date? It is not expired milk, it is more like cheese; it gets funkier, richer and occasionally smells suspicious, but it is worth savoring. We are not on a countdown to irrelevance. We are on a lifelong road trip, complete with detours, snack breaks, and the occasional "What was

I saying again?" moment. And if you are lucky, you reach the glorious phase where you stop caring about what anyone thinks and start wearing leopard print without irony.

Instead of asking people to "act their age," maybe we should be asking what they feel like doing today; be it starting a podcast, joining a hip-hop class or finally telling Cheryl from HR that yes, they can use Excel, and in fact, invented the spreadsheet during the Reagan administration.

Let us quit acting like age is the problem. The real issue is a society trying to shove everyone into neat little boxes marked "young and clueless" or "old and obsolete." Here is a newsflash: people contain multitudes. You can be a grandmother and a gamer, a retiree and a rapper, a twenty-year-old who loves tea and cardigans or a seventy-year-old who rollerblades to punk rock. Age does not define us; it just adds more chapters to the story.

We should long ago have thrown the age rulebook out with the floppy disks. Let us celebrate the glorious chaos of a world where a 19-year-old and a 91-year-old can both go viral, where every age comes with its own brand of brilliance, and where the only real limitation is assuming there is a "right" time to be anything. After all, life is a potluck, and everyone's dish matters, whether it is wisdom, weird dance moves, or just showing up with snacks.

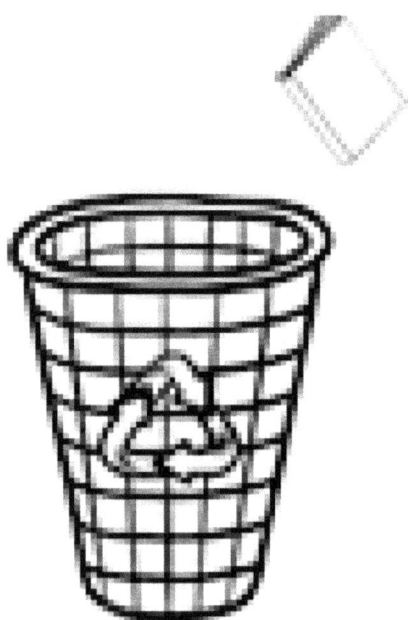

Chapter 5:

The Impact of Technology

Old Dogs, New Clicks: Aging Gracefully with Innovations Enhanced Longevity

Welcome to the digital age, where your cellphone is smarter than you are, where your refrigerator talks back, and where your grandchild insists that "it is all in the cloud," which, frankly, sounds like a storage unit guarded by a unicorn. For those who remember life before email, it is a little like being dropped into a high-speed video game without the cheat codes. But if you can survive dial-up, floppy disks, and that one time you accidentally set your VCR to record six months of golf, you can definitely survive this.

Technology now runs our lives or at least jogs beside us shouting "update required!" We order coffee through apps, find love (or something like it) via swipes, and ghost people without leaving the house. And every time we figure it out, someone moves the "send" button, changes the password rules, or invents a new platform that sounds like a sneeze. X? Telegram? Threads? My goodness, it is starting to feel like social media is an exam we did not study for.

Age is not a handicap here; it is a secret weapon. You have already outlived landlines and MySpace. You know what a fax machine is. That kind of resilience should come with a cape.

The digital world may be fast, flashy, and full of acronyms, but it is also wide open for curious minds. You can learn Portuguese at midnight, master the ukulele by Tuesday, and Google just about anything from how to change a tire to "What is Bitcoin and why does it sound like pirate treasure?"

Best of all, technology has turned into a surprise family reunion planner. Grandma can attend dinner via Zoom (even if she is accidentally live-streaming the ceiling), and Grandpa can post memes about "back in my day" while the grandchildren pretend not to know him in the comment section. It is chaotic, yes, but it is connection, albeit filtered, pixelated, and occasionally upside down.

Digital life is not all rainbows and free Wi-Fi. Some of us still treat our email inbox like a haunted attic that we are too afraid to open. And let us not talk about the terrifying moment when you realize you just posted your late-night rash search on Facebook. But even these missteps are badges of honor. We are not failing; we are learning with style and maybe a few typos.

And if you think aging and technology do not mix, think again. Scientists are rewriting the rules on what it means to grow older. Aging used to mean accepting the slow creak of your joints and becoming best friends with your heating pad. Now, it is all about stem cells, wearables, AI-powered wellness apps and nutrition that promises immortality (or at least fewer naps).

Stem cell therapies are like spa days for your cells, gently whispering, "You can do this. You are still young-ish." Artificial

Intelligence (AI) plays the role of a cheerful health nerd who keeps tabs on your blood pressure and gently suggests you skip that fourth glass of red. We have even reached the point where kale is pretending to be candy and smartwatches are tattling on you for skipping your steps.

Welcome to the future, where your salad judges you and your fridge sends you texts. But underneath all this innovation the message is simple: aging is not about fading out; it is about leaning in. The goal is not just to live longer, but to live louder. We are not relics; we are Renaissance 2.0. And whether you are embracing technology with open arms or cautiously poking it with a stylus, the truth is this: you are part of the upgrade.

So here is to a life filled with curious clicks, a few digital blunders, and the kind of joy that only comes from mixing a little wisdom with a lot of Wi-Fi.

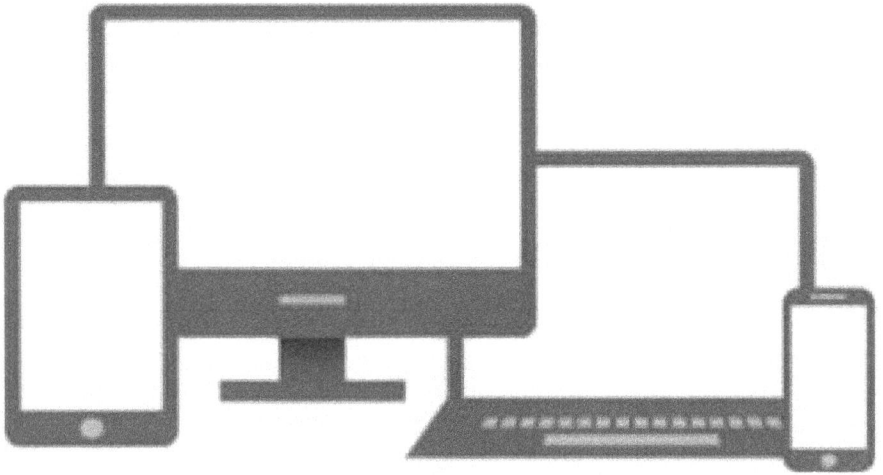

I do not need a relationship. I just want someone who understands my browser history and doesn't judge me.

Chapter 6:

Redefining Milestones

How to ignore the Manual and still win the Game of Life

Once upon a time, life came with a pretty rigid to-do list: graduate, get a job, marry someone reasonably tolerable, have children, buy a house, and eventually retire somewhere warm to complain about the youth. These days, that list has been shredded, set on fire, and replaced with a messy but glorious buffet of choices, detours, and "wait, what am I doing?" moments.

Forget age brackets and timelines. Life stages in the 21st century are more like jazz; unpredictable, occasionally chaotic, and best enjoyed when you stop trying to control the tempo. Education is not just for the young anymore. Fifty-year-olds are going back to school, not to relive their glory days but because they finally want to understand quantum physics, graphic design, or how to use Midjourney without starting a technical support group.

Adulthood, that elusive state we were all promised would bring stability and answers, turns out to be more of a DIY project with no instructions and missing screws. Some folks are starting businesses in their thirties, others are finding themselves on silent yoga retreats in their fifties, and a few are just now realizing avocado toast does not qualify as a personality.

Middle age used to mean "over the hill," but now it is more like "over the moon with new hobbies." It is the golden era of reinvention. People are buying motorbikes, writing screenplays, taking up kung fu, or mastering the art of baking sourdough bread like it is an Olympic sport. It is less crisis and more comeback tour but with better lighting and a lot more turmeric.

And then we have the so-called golden years, which are no longer about slowing down but leveling up. Retirement looks less like bingo and more like building empires, becoming internet-famous for your baking skills, or running marathons with knees that somehow still work. Grandparents today do not just hand out Werther's Originals. They are giving TED Talks, climbing mountains and learning to create digital art that leaves their grandchildren slightly horrified but secretly impressed.

Personal growth is a state of mind, and it is not just for the fresh-faced and flexible anymore. It is for the curious, the brave, and those who finally decide to face their fear of Pilates head-on (or head-down, depending on the pose). Whether it is finally sorting your emotional baggage or learning to ask for help without muttering through gritted teeth, evolving is the new sexy. Think of it as software updates for your soul with fewer bugs and better emotional bandwidth.

Recognizing achievements, big or small, is also a secret sauce for feeling good about yourself. Whether it is conquering a fear or just remembering where you left your glasses, every win boosts confidence and lights the path to new adventures. Life is not a sprint to impress strangers; it is a marathon of celebrating those moments that make you smile and maybe occasionally dance like no one is watching.

Success is not one-size-fits-all. It is a mismatched, slightly chaotic wardrobe of milestones: learning to cook something that does not involve a microwave, finally remembering what that button on the remote does, or launching your side hustle in your sixties just because you can. When we toss out the traditional checklist and make room for quirky, beautiful progress, we create a world where everyone's growth is valid and celebrated. These wins may not come with trophies, but they deserve their own victory laps.

So, raise a glass (or a green smoothie, if that is your vibe) to rewriting the playbook. The best part is that you are the author now. And in this version, there is no such thing as being "too late" only right on time with better stories and great dance moves to show for it. When we cheer each other's unique journeys, we build a culture that is far more fun, inclusive and inspiring, because the best accomplishments are the ones that make you feel alive, no matter what the calendar says.

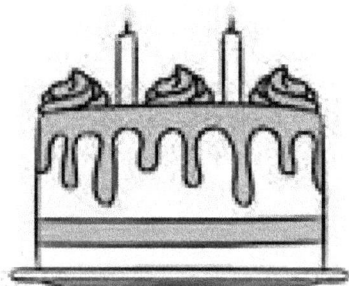

Celebrate until even your
confetti needs a nap

Chapter 7:

Intergenerational Relationships

Bridging the Generation Gap and Learning from Each Other

In a world obsessed with categories such as vegan or carnivore, iPhone or Android, Spotify or "what's streaming," age is just another label we love to overuse. But peel back the layers of gray hair and YouTube trends and you will find something beautifully simple: we have stories, strengths, and at least one embarrassing moment we can laugh about together. Bridging the so-called generation gap is less about building bridges and more about realizing there was never really a canyon in the first place, just some mismatched slang and questionable fashion choices.

When different age groups sit down and talk (preferably with snacks), something magical happens. The young bring their wide-eyed optimism, technical skills, and baffling text speak. The older generation contributes experience, resilience and the rare ability to sit through an entire phone conversation without Googling something halfway through. The result is mutual admiration, occasional confusion, and a lot of wisdom flying in both directions.

Forget the idea that only the young teach the old. These days, it is a two-way street with surprisingly good traffic flow. Younger folks help seniors decode the mysteries of Bluetooth, while older folks teach patience by not throttling anyone mid-tech tutorial. Schools, libraries, and community groups are catching on to this power combo, inviting people of all ages to mingle, learn, and occasionally mispronounce each other's slang.

And then there is the magic of stories. Nothing connects generations like a good tale, whether it is Grandma recalling the drama of dial-up internet or a teenager navigating life through memes. These stories are sticky. They burrow into hearts, broaden minds, and prove that even if your music tastes clash like plaid and polka dots, your experiences might just harmonize perfectly.

Community is where all this comes to life. A real community is not just about waving at your neighbor once every three months; it is about knowing you have a go-to crew for everything from cookie recipes to life advice. It is where "I have been through that" meets "I had no idea," and both sides walk away feeling smarter, stronger, and more seen. Age does not divide us here; it enriches the mix. Because nothing beats sharing a laugh, a memory, or a cup of tea with someone who sees the world just a little differently.

Life moves fast, but if we pause long enough to listen, learn, and lean in, we discover that we are all just trying to make sense of this wonderfully weird ride together. The generation gap is more like a hop, skip, and a shared playlist away. When we ditch the stereotypes and show up with curiosity (and maybe muffins), we turn age into an asset, not a divider. And that is the secret to keeping life full of connection, purpose, and just the right amount of sparkle no matter what your birth certificate says.

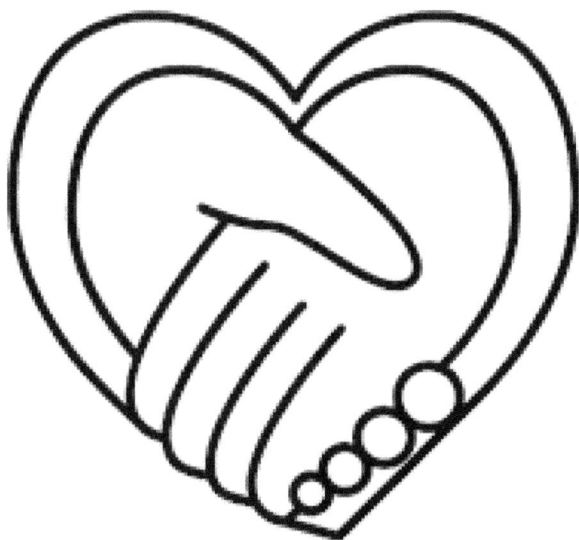

Chapter 8:

The Role of Purpose

Every Decade Has Got Its Own Drama (and Glory)

Every decade brings its own brand of drama, wonder, and occasional back pain. Our twenties are full of energy and indecision like being dropped into a buffet with no instructions, where everything looks delicious, but you are not quite sure what will give you indigestion. It is a time of discovery, bold dreams, and the kind of choices that make for great stories later or cautionary tales.

Then come the years when multitasking becomes a competitive sport, juggling work, relationships, identity and taxes without dropping the ball or at least pretending we did not turn it into an art form. Somewhere between climbing career ladders and forgetting why we walked into a room, we start asking deeper questions: What really matters? Is this it? Should I take up pottery?

By the time we reach the fifties and sixties, something shifts. There is less performing and more being. You have earned the right to care less about what others think and more about what truly brings you joy. You ask yourself if you should revitalize that project you shelved, or what changes you should make to your usual weekend activities. And oddly enough, you are starting to believe you really might write that novel after all or start astrology lessons maybe even on the same day.

Later in life, the spotlight moves from proving yourself to enjoying yourself. It is about being present for the small things, such as a proper cup of tea, a walk without a deadline, or the luxury of retelling your best anecdotes without shame. It is less about goals and more about grace. And those stories you tell become less about you alone and more about offering a gift to others, a legacy in motion.

"Purpose" does not come with a manual or a deadline. It is less about climbing mountains and more about choosing which view to admire. Everyone has something valuable to give, from the young who might offer ideas so fast you need subtitles, to the older who know things Google does not. When generations join forces, whether through conversation, collaboration or a shared Spotify playlist, they create communities that thrive, full of depth, humor and an unusual number of snacks.

"Meaning" is not reserved for the famous or the fearless. It lives in quiet acts of kindness, in stories told over dinner and in wisdom passed down when no one is looking. A legacy is not built in a day; it is stitched together from countless ordinary moments made extraordinary by care, connection and a dash of boldness.

The beauty of purpose is that it evolves. What drives you in your twenties will not be what moves you in your seventies and that is the point. Life is an ever-changing plotline, and the goal is not to stick to the script but to keep showing up for the next scene, preferably with popcorn.

Chapter 9:

Health and Well-being (with a wink and a stretch)

Holistic Approaches to Aging: Because we are More Than Just Achy Knees

Aging could really use a better spin doctor. The narrative is all creaky joints, memory lapses and a slow shuffle into obscurity. But we are not falling apart; we are just evolving with a few more sound effects. The truth is that there is nothing "less than" about growing older. We are not just a collection of aches and medication reminders; we are full-bodied, full-spirited humans with sharp minds, rich experience, and the occasional misplacement of our spectacles (check your head). This is not the countdown phase; it is the glow-up.

Holistic aging is less about denying time and more about owning it. It is the deluxe version of self-care, where your mind, body, and soul get equal billing. Mental well-being is not a luxury, it is essential. Think of creativity, hobbies and lifelong learning as brain snacks. Meditation might sound like something Gwyneth Paltrow whispers over a candle, but it actually works, lower stress, better sleep and fewer irrational urges to yell at your plants.

To maintain physical health, you do not need to join a CrossFit cult. A brisk walk, a casual boogie in the kitchen, a little gardening drama with a rebellious zucchini. Movement counts no matter how it looks with bonus points if it involves giggling. Add any food that actually nourishes you such as fruits, vegetables, and yes, the occasional donut to maintain your emotional balance and you are basically a vintage Rolls Royce with excellent mileage.

Do not underestimate the magic of human connection either. Aging is way more fun with co-conspirators. Whether it is book clubs, quiz nights, or long chats over coffee that veer off into laughing fits, community is the invisible vitamin. You might be aging, but you are not meant to do it solo. We thrive in company, preferably the kind that texts you memes and knows when you need a hug or a cocktail.

Of course, mental health does not politely excuse itself just because you have reached a certain age. Emotional challenges might pop up, such as grief, loneliness and anxiety, but so do surprising pockets of peace and clarity. You finally have time to think your thoughts all the way through. Therapy and journaling are absolutely helpful and recommended. But crying over a touching dog commercial just means you have a lovely heart or perhaps that is just called Tuesday. Let us normalize asking for help and talking it out. You would not ignore a weird rattle in your car, so do not ignore one in your chest.

The point is that aging well is not about clinging to youth; it is about leaning into your present with both arms, a sense of humor and a good moisturizer. It is about getting up (slowly), showing up (with snacks) and laughing often (ideally until you snort). You are not past your prime, you have just entered the director's cut.

You do not need to be a kale-smoothie-sipping yoga master or a marathon-running meditation guru. You just need to move a little, eat what feels good, talk to people who make you feel alive and embrace the beautiful absurdity of it all. Your laugh lines are a flex and your quirks are trademarks. You are not over the hill; you are the hill, and it has a stunning view.

Let us make sure everyone gets to age with joy, with dignity and preferably with someone to split dessert with.

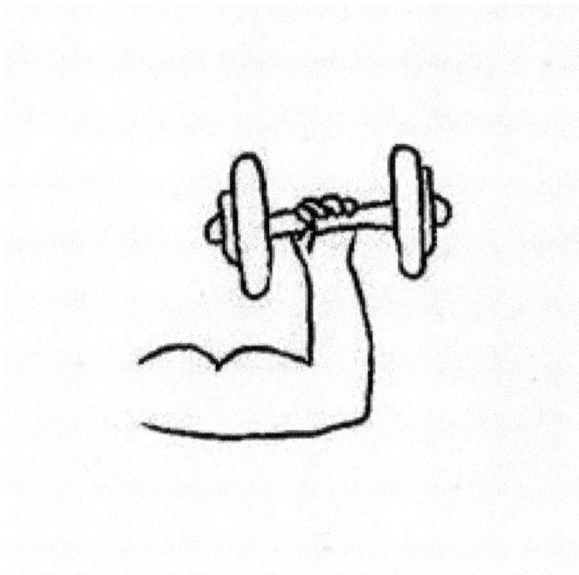

Chapter 10:
The Future of Aging
Where Age Is Just Your Wi-Fi Password Recovery Question

Picture a world where no one blinks if a 92-year-old joins a breakdancing class or a teenager hosts a podcast called "Tea with Granny." In this future, age is not something to whisper about or camouflage with oversized sunglasses. It is a plot twist, not a plot end. Life does not politely step aside after 60, instead, it moonwalks into new careers, side hustles and possibly salsa lessons. You are never "too old" to start over, you are just seasoned enough to skip the rookie mistakes.

Forget the tired narrative of slowing down with age. This new chapter comes with speed bumps, and yes, even turbo boosters. Education does not retire, it reboots. Whether you are keen on black holes or just trying to escape your own digital inbox, learning is always on the menu, served with both kombucha and a custard tart, depending on your era.

Society should stop acting like it is at a high school dance where generations stick to their own corners. Instead, we all mix playlists, life hacks and recipes; TikTok meets Tupperware. NFTs share shelf space with VHS tapes. We celebrate the curious toddler and the curious retiree because one is learning to walk and the other to moonwalk. Technology is no longer a battleground between "back in my day" and "what even is a landline?" Everyone learns from everyone. Grandpa can FaceTime. Gen Alpha knows how to sew on a button (well, we are working on that). And yes, someone will finally explain blockchain in a way that does not make it sound like a medical condition.

We build communities that do not just accommodate, they anticipate from shared housing across age groups to workplace teams that combine the wisdom of experience with the audacity of youth. The future gets things done with flair and probably a group chat named "Silver and Sassy."

And let us not forget attitude. This future society laughs in the face of age-based limits. "You are too old for that" gets the same treatment as dot-matrix printers: unplugged and tossed out. We should stop measuring life by milestones and start measuring it by moments like the time your grandmother went viral for her unboxing video or when your intern taught you to code and crochet in the same afternoon. Whether it is war stories, rave stories or just a shared obsession with oat milk and crossword puzzles, we need each other.

Here is your call to action, wrapped in a warm hug and maybe a reusable shopping bag:

- Speak up.

- Link arms across generations.

- Start projects that span ages and Spotify playlists.

- And, most importantly, do not wait to be invited to the party. Be the one who brings the chicken wings, the playlist, and a bingo board, just in case.

In this worldwide vision of timeless societies, aging is not something to fear; it is something to celebrate. Like a well-aged wine or a legendary leather jacket, we only get more interesting with time. Let us build this future together. Wrinkles are earned, wisdom is shared and nobody gets left behind because of the date on their driver's license. After all, we are not aging; we are just getting better at being "us". The future is not just young, it is ageless, and it has a great sense of humor.

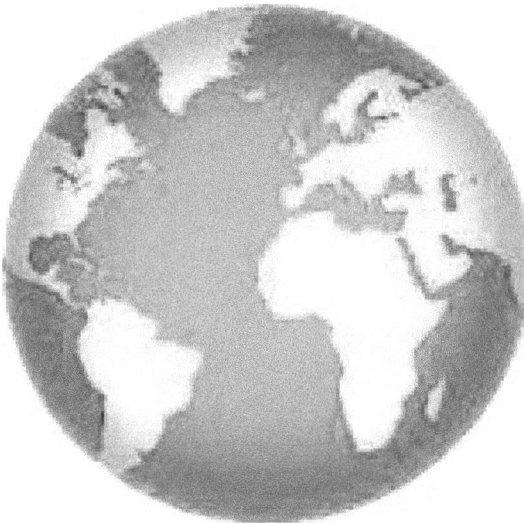